I0781969

The 2024 Complete Vaginal Candidiasis Guide

Understanding Vaginal Candidiasis, Yeast
Infection Symptoms, Causes and
Treatments for Beginners

Elizabeth A. Bragg

Copyright 2024

Elizabeth A. Bragg. All rights reserved.

No part of this book may be copied, distributed, or transmitted in any way without the author's prior written consent; the only exceptions are brief quotations included in critical reviews and certain other noncommercial uses allowed by copyright law. This includes photocopying, recording, and other electronic or mechanical methods.

DISCLAIMER !!!

This book contains information that should only be used for educational and informational reasons; it is not meant to be used as medical advice. The information provided does not replace a qualified medical professional's diagnosis, care, or counsel. Always consult your doctor or another licensed healthcare professional with any questions you may have about a medical condition or course of treatment.

The accuracy, applicability, and completeness of the information in this book are not warranted or represented by the author or publisher. The use or misuse of the material included in this book may result in injury, loss, or damage, for which the author assumes no responsibility. Before starting any new medication, diet, or fitness regimen, the reader should speak with a healthcare professional. The reader is ultimately accountable for their own health decisions.

This book's material should be understood as such, as it is based on the author's personal experiences, research, and opinions. Since the medical world is always changing, new material may become available that surpasses the information in this book. For the most recent information, the author advises readers to stay educated and to seek advice from professionals and reliable sources.

Table of content

Introduction

Yeast infections, or vaginal candidiasis, are a frequent medical issue that affects millions of women worldwide. The overabundance of Candida yeast in the vaginal region is the reason, resulting in symptoms like burning, itching, and strange discharge. Even though it's a frequent problem, the misery and shame that come with it can be unbearable, therefore it's important to fully grasp the situation.

The goal of this book is to give readers a thorough overview of vaginal candidiasis, including information on its causes, symptoms, successful treatments, and preventative measures. Whether this is your first infection or you're struggling with recurrent episodes, this book will provide you with the information and resources you need to effectively manage and avoid this condition.

As 2024 draws to a close, the field of women's health is still changing quickly due to the rapid development of new knowledge, therapies, and perspectives. Although vaginal candidiasis is still a common problem, management and prevention strategies have greatly improved. For women who want to take charge of their health, this guide is a timely resource because it includes the most recent knowledge and techniques.

Apart from modern medical interventions, the significance of complementary and preventative care is being increasingly recognized. This manual combines traditional and natural methods, understanding that each woman's body is distinct and may react differently to different therapies.

This book gives you the tools to make well-informed decisions about your health that are customized to meet your own needs by providing a balanced viewpoint.

Whether you are new to the subject or have had yeast infections for years, this book is meant to help you better understand vaginal candidiasis. It is particularly useful for:

Women with their first yeast infection: This information will help you understand what you have, how to treat it, and how to avoid being infected again if you're new to vaginal candidiasis.

Those with recurring infections: This book provides information on why yeast infections might be happening again and how to stop the cycle if you've had several infections.

Medical practitioners: This handbook is a useful tool for patient education for physicians, nurses, and other healthcare professionals. It provides concise explanations and helpful guidance.

Carers and partners: This book will help you better understand vaginal candidiasis so that you may provide knowledgeable and understanding support to someone who has the illness.

To treat present infections, avert future ones, or just increase your understanding of women's health, this handbook provides the most up-to-date, thorough, and useful information about women's health that will be accessible in 2024.

Chapter One

Getting to Know Vaginal Candida

What Is Candida in the Vagina?

A yeast infection, also known as vaginal candidiasis, is a fungal infection caused by an overabundance of Candida yeast in the vaginal region. One form of yeast that occurs naturally in small amounts in the mouth, stomach, and vagina is called Candida. In healthy conditions, beneficial bacteria and the immune system of the body suppress the growth of Candida. But if these microbes' delicate equilibrium is upset, Candida may proliferate uncontrollably and cause infection.

Intense itching, burning, swelling, and a thick, white discharge that resembles cottage cheese are some of the symptoms of vaginal candidiasis. Millions of women suffer from this common ailment, but if left untreated, it can be extremely uncomfortable and result in more serious issues.

The Candida Overgrowth's Science

Studying the science of Candida proliferation is crucial to understanding vaginal candidiasis. One kind of yeast that is a member of the fungal kingdom is called Candida. Although Candida comes in many different species, Candida albicans is the most frequently linked species to vaginal infections.

Candida coexists in a healthy vagina with other microorganisms, including Lactobacillus and other helpful bacteria that contribute to the acidic environment that prevents the formation of pathogenic species. But several things have the potential to upset this delicate equilibrium and cause Candida overgrowth:

By eliminating good bacteria in the vagina, antibiotics can promote the growth of Candida.

An environment that is favorable to yeast overgrowth can be produced by fluctuations in hormone levels, such as those that happen during pregnancy, menstruation, or as a result of using hormonal contraceptives.

The body's capacity to regulate Candida growth may be weakened by an immune system that is weakened as a result of disease, stress, or certain drugs.

Women with uncontrolled diabetes are more vulnerable to vaginal candidiasis because high blood sugar can encourage the growth of yeast in the body.

Comprehending these variables is essential for both prophylaxis and therapy since tackling the underlying reason for Candida hypergrowth can aid in controlling and diminishing the likelihood of subsequent infections.

Vaginal Infection Types:
Bacterial Vaginosis vs Candidiasis

Despite being one of the most prevalent vaginal diseases, vaginal candidiasis must be distinguished from other infections, especially bacterial vaginosis (BV). While there are certain symptoms common to both illnesses, their causes and therapies are distinct.

- **Vaginal Candidiasis:** Candida yeast overgrowth is the cause of vaginal candidiasis, as was previously mentioned. It usually manifests as burning, itching, and a thick, white discharge.

- **Bacterial Vaginosis (BV):** An excess of pathogenic bacteria results from a disruption in the normal balance of microorganisms in the vagina. BV is a bacterial illness. Symptoms of bacterial vaginosis (BV) include a thin, fishy-smelling discharge that is grayish-white in color and differs from those of yeast infections.

The two illnesses' causes and symptoms are where the main distinctions between them are found. Both can be uncomfortable and disruptive, but they need to be treated differently. Comprehending these distinctions is imperative for accurate diagnosis and treatment planning, guaranteeing that the appropriate therapy is administered to reinstate vaginal health.

Understanding the causes, symptoms, and distinctions between vaginal candidiasis and other frequent vaginal infections will help you recognize the illness's symptoms early and seek appropriate treatment. Gaining this understanding is the first step to managing your vaginal health and averting more infections.

Chapter Two

Vaginal Candidiasis Symptoms

Yeast infections, also referred to as vaginal candidiasis, can cause a range of symptoms, from moderate to severe. Early diagnosis and treatment can help you avoid more agony and seek help as soon as possible. Among the most typical symptoms are:

Itching and Irritation: The main signs of a yeast infection are persistent itching and irritation in the vulvar and vaginal regions. Extreme itching can cause discomfort and even interfere with day-to-day activities.

Burning Sensation: During sexual activity or urination, many women report feeling as though they are being burned. This may indicate that the vaginal tissues have become inflamed due to the infection.

Unusual Vaginal Discharge: Another typical symptom is a thick, clumpy, white discharge that resembles cottage cheese. This, in contrast to regular discharge, is often odorless but occasionally has a sour scent to it.

Redness and Swelling: The infection-related inflammation may cause the vulva to seem red, swollen, and sensitive.

Soreness and Pain: Sitting, walking, and having sex can be painful for some women due to soreness or pain in the vaginal area.

Although these are common signs of vaginal candidiasis, each individual may experience these symptoms differently in terms of strength and combination.

How to Tell the Difference Between Other Infections and Candidiasis

Though prevalent, vaginal candidiasis might have symptoms that are similar to other vaginal infections; therefore, it's necessary to distinguish between the two to receive the right therapy. Here's how to tell candidiasis apart from other prevalent infections:

Bacterial Vaginosis (BV): Because of its comparable symptoms, such as discomfort and itching, BV is sometimes confused with a yeast infection. On the other hand, BV-related discharge is usually thin, white, or grayish-white, and smells strongly of fish. Yeast infection discharge, on the other hand, is typically thick, white, and odorless.

Trichomoniasis: This STI may present with burning and itching sensations akin to those of a yeast infection. However, unlike the discharge seen with candidiasis, trichomoniasis frequently creates a frothy, yellow-green discharge with an unpleasant smell.

Urinary Tract Infection (UTI): Symptoms of a UTI include burning when urinating, frequent urination, and lower abdomen pain. UTIs mostly affect the urinary system. While vaginal itching and discharge associated with candidiasis are usually not caused by UTIs, yeast infections can produce a burning feeling.

Contact Dermatitis: This ailment is brought on by an allergic response to or irritation from materials such as clothes, detergents, or soaps. It lacks the discharge common to candidiasis and is typically associated with the use of a new product. It can induce itching and redness comparable to a yeast infection.

A trip to the doctor is frequently necessary for a proper diagnosis, particularly if symptoms are new to you or if over-the-counter remedies aren't helping.

<u>When to Get Medical Assistance</u>

Even though many women may treat moderate yeast infections with over-the-counter medications, there are some circumstances in which seeing a doctor is crucial:

Recurrent Infections: A yeast infection is deemed recurrent if it occurs more than four times in a calendar year. This can point to a more serious problem that requires medical care.

Severe Symptoms: It is preferable to speak with a healthcare professional about stronger or prescription-strength remedies if your symptoms are severe, such as severe itching, noticeable swelling, or sores.

Uncertain Diagnosis: To make sure you're receiving the appropriate therapy, it's critical to receive a professional diagnosis if you're not sure if your symptoms are caused by a yeast infection or something else.

Pregnancy: You must see a doctor if you think you may have a yeast infection while pregnant. Although yeast infections are frequent during pregnancy, special care is needed to prevent problems.

Lack of Improvement: You should consult a doctor if, after using over-the-counter remedies, your symptoms have not improved or have gotten worse in a few days.

Getting medical attention as soon as possible will help avoid problems and guarantee that you get the best care possible for your illness. Recall that while yeast infections are frequent, you shouldn't ignore them, particularly if they worsen or become recurring.

Chapter Three

Vaginal Candidiasis Causes

An overabundance of Candida yeast, especially Candida albicans, in the vaginal region results in vaginal candidiasis. This overgrowth may be caused by several things, upsetting the normal balance of microorganisms:

Hormonal Changes: Candida may flourish in an environment where there are fluctuations in hormone levels, such as those brought on by hormonal contraceptives, menstruation, or pregnancy. For example, elevated estrogen levels can encourage the growth of yeast.

Weakened Immune System: Immunosuppressive drugs, chronic illnesses, or diseases can all weaken the immune system, making it more difficult for the body to regulate the overgrowth of Candida.

Excessive Blood Sugar Levels: Yeast growth can be fuelled by uncontrolled diabetes or excessive blood sugar levels. Candida is a yeast that grows well in sweet conditions, and high blood sugar levels give the yeast an abundance of resources.

Increased Moisture and Heat: Candida can develop in moist, heated settings, such as those produced by tight or airtight garments. For this reason, hot, muggy weather tends to increase the prevalence of yeast infections.

Stress: Extended periods of stress can impair hormone balance and erode immunity, leaving the body more vulnerable to infections, including yeast infections.

Diet and Lifestyle's Significance

Vaginal health is greatly influenced by diet and lifestyle decisions, which can also affect the risk of vaginal candidiasis:

Diet High in Refined Carbs and Sugar: Eating a diet high in refined carbs and sugar can cause an overgrowth of yeast. Since *Candida* feeds on sugar, consuming a lot of these items can increase the growth of the yeast.

Deficiency in Probiotics: Probiotics, which are present in foods like yogurt and fermented goods, assist in preserving the body's natural microbiota balance. An imbalance that promotes yeast growth can result from a lack of probiotics.

Improper Hygiene Practices: Douching, wearing non-breathable pants, and using scented hygiene products can upset the vagina's natural pH balance and promote yeast overgrowth. Infections can be avoided by practicing good hygiene and using gentle, odorless products.

Sexual Activity: Unprotected or frequent sex can spread new bacteria into the vaginal region, increasing the risk of infection. Yeast infections, however, are not considered sexually transmitted infections in and of themselves.

Drugs and Their Effects on the Health of the Vagina

Certain drugs may have an impact on vaginal health and may even cause vaginal candidiasis to develop:

Antibiotics: By eliminating the good bacteria that inhibit Candida, antibiotics might upset the normal bacterial balance in the vagina. This disturbance may cause yeast to overgrow.

Hormonal Medications: Birth control pills and hormone replacement therapy are examples of hormonal contraceptives that might alter hormone levels and possibly exacerbate yeast overgrowth.

Immunosuppressive Drugs: Drugs that suppress the immune system, including corticosteroids or chemotherapy, can lessen the body's capacity to regulate the growth of Candida, which raises the risk of infections.

Steroid Creams: Using topical steroid creams in the genital area over an extended period might change the vaginal environment and impair local immunity, which can result in yeast infections.

Knowing About Recurrent Infections

Recurrent vaginal candidiasis is characterized by four or more infections during 12 months. Effective management of recurring illnesses requires an understanding of their underlying causes:

Chronic Conditions: People who suffer from diabetes or autoimmune diseases are more likely to get yeast infections frequently. To stop recurrence, these underlying problems must be managed.

Incomplete Treatment: If an over-the-counter medicine is used inappropriately or if a prescribed antifungal medication is not finished in its entirety, the infection may not be completely eradicated, which could lead to recurrence.

Partner Transmission: While not considered a sexually transmitted infection, vaginal candidiasis can occasionally be carried by and shared between partners. Recurrence can be decreased by making sure that both couples receive treatment when required.

Lifestyle Factors: Recurrent infections can be caused by chronic lifestyle factors such as an unhealthy diet, excessive levels of stress, or improper hygiene practices. Preventing future incidents requires addressing these factors.

The therapy and prevention of vaginal candidiasis can both benefit from an understanding of these causes and contributory variables. People can better control and lower the risk of recurrent infections by recognizing and resolving these concerns.

Chapter Four

Vaginal Candida Diagnosis Diagnosis

Methods for Diagnosing Vaginal Candidiasis

Lab testing and clinical assessment are usually used in the diagnosis of vaginal candidiasis. This is a detailed flowchart of the diagnostic procedure:

Medical History and Symptoms: Talking with a healthcare professional about your medical history and symptoms is the first step. They'll enquire about the type of symptoms you're experiencing, how long they've lasted, and any potential triggers. This aids in separating the infection-type candidiasis from others.

Physical Examination: To evaluate the state of the vaginal tissues, a physical examination, which includes a pelvic exam, is typically performed. The healthcare practitioner will be on the lookout for discharge, edema, and redness.

Microscopic Examination: During the pelvic exam, a sample of vaginal discharge may be taken and studied under a microscope. This could indicate that you have a yeast infection if Candida cells or hyphae (fungal components) are present.

Culture Test: To develop and identify the particular strain of Candida, a culture of the vaginal discharge may occasionally be obtained. This is especially helpful if the illness recurs or if conventional therapy is ineffective in treating the symptoms.

pH Testing: A vaginal pH test can be used to distinguish between various infections and candidiasis. Typically, the pH of the vagina is acidic, ranging from 3.8 to 4.5. While trichomoniasis or bacterial vaginosis frequently causes a higher pH, candidiasis usually does not affect the vaginal pH.

Home Test Kits: Benefits and Drawbacks

Vaginal infection testing kits can be purchased over-the-counter and provide a handy means of evaluating your symptoms. But they have benefits and drawbacks as well:

Positives:

- Convenience: Tests at home can be conducted quickly and discreetly; a visit to the doctor is not necessary. Those looking for quick fixes may find this especially enticing.

Cost-Effective: For some people, home testing kits are a more affordable option than seeing a healthcare professional because they are frequently less expensive.

- Early Detection: By identifying possible infections early, these tests can help you seek professional medical care as soon as possible.

Drawbacks:

Accuracy: Compared to professional diagnostic techniques, home tests might not be as reliable. False positives or false negatives can happen, which can result in an inaccurate self-diagnosis and ineffective care.

- **Limited Scope:** Although home kits usually check for the presence of Candida, they might not be able to distinguish between various illnesses or pinpoint underlying problems.

- **No Professional Guidance:** A comprehensive evaluation or professional medical advice is not provided by home testing. If the test is positive, this may lead to a lack of direction regarding the next course of action.

Misinterpretation: There's a chance of misinterpreting the results and postponing necessary therapy if a healthcare professional isn't there to interpret them.

<u>The Significance of a Qualified Diagnosis</u>

Although home testing kits might offer initial insights, seeking a professional diagnosis is imperative for multiple reasons:

- **Accurate Diagnosis:** A medical professional is qualified to identify vaginal candidiasis and distinguish it from other infections or illnesses that may exhibit comparable symptoms.

- **Appropriate Treatment:** Having a professional diagnosis guarantees that the best care is given for your particular ailment. Prescription drugs or a mix of therapies may be used in this.

- **Comprehensive Care:** Medical professionals can assess your general state of health and pinpoint any underlying causes of recurrent infections. They can also address any worries you may have and offer guidance on lifestyle modifications and preventative actions.

Follow-Up: If symptoms worsen or return, a medical professional may recommend further testing or, if necessary, send you to a specialist.

Prevention of Complications: Careful assessment and diagnosis aid in avoiding possible problems or improper treatment of the ailment. This is especially crucial in cases of severe symptoms or infections that keep coming back.

convenient home testing kits shouldn't take the place of a qualified medical examination. For vaginal candidiasis to be correctly identified, effectively treated, and given thorough care, a healthcare provider's diagnosis is crucial.

Chapter Five

Typical Vaginal Candidiasis Treatments

Off-the-Counter Medication

When treating vaginal candidiasis, over-the-counter (OTC) medications are frequently the primary line of treatment, particularly in instances that are not too difficult. These treatments, which are easily obtained without a prescription, consist of:

Antifungal Creams: Direct application of over-the-counter antifungal creams, such as those containing miconazole or clotrimazole, to the afflicted area is recommended. By eliminating the yeast, these treatments reduce burning and itchy sensations.

Suppositories: Miconazole or tioconazole-containing vaginal suppositories are placed into the vagina. With time, they dissolve and release the antifungal drug to fight the infection.

Ointments: To ease itching and discomfort around the vulva, certain over-the-counter medications are available as topically administered ointments.

Over-the-counter medications are easily acquired and frequently offer prompt relief from mild infections. Compared to prescription drugs, they are typically less expensive.

Over-the-counter (OTC) medicines may not be efficacious in treating severe or recurrent illnesses, nor do they address the root causes. You run the risk of misdiagnosing the infection and treating it improperly in the absence of a professional diagnosis.

Medication Prescriptions

Prescription drugs might be required for cases of vaginal candidiasis that are more severe or recurrent. Among them are:

Oral Antifungals: Fluconazole (Diflucan) and other oral medications are useful in treating more serious or recurrent infections. They function by preventing Candida from spreading throughout the body.

Topical Antifungals: If over-the-counter remedies don't work for more severe cases, prescription-strength topical medications may be utilized. These consist of ointments, suppositories, and creams that have stronger antifungal agent concentrations.

For severe or chronic infections, prescription drugs are frequently more effective. Depending on the strain of Candida and the extent of the infection, a medical professional can recommend the best course of action. Prescription drugs might be more costly than over-the-counter alternatives.

To ensure appropriate diagnosis and treatment, a prescription must be evaluated by a healthcare provider.

<u>The Function of Tablets and Creams Antifungal</u>

Since they specifically target the Candida yeast, antifungal therapies are essential for the management of vaginal candidiasis. Oral and topical antifungals have different applications.

- **Topical Antifungals:** These include creams, ointments, and suppositories that are applied directly to the afflicted area. For simple infections, they usually work well and offer localized treatment. By getting rid of yeast from the vaginal tissues, they relieve discomfort.

- **Oral Antifungals:** More serious or recurring infections are treated with oral drugs like fluconazole. They treat the infection systemically, which means they don't only target it locally. These are particularly helpful if the infection is extensive or topical therapies are not enough.

Combining topical and oral antifungals can yield better results when treating complicated cases.

Both varieties of antifungals aid in the removal of infection-causing yeast and the alleviation of symptoms. Adhering to the recommended dosage and duration is crucial for both preventing resistance and ensuring an effective course of therapy. To guarantee appropriate use and efficacy, a healthcare professional should give guidance when using these treatments.

Possible Adverse Reactions to Conventional Therapy

Conventional treatments have the potential for negative effects even while they are effective:

Topical Antifungals: Burning, redness, or local irritation at the application site are possible side effects. Usually minor, these side effects go away on their own after the medication is stopped.

Oral Antifungals: Medications used orally may have systemic side effects, including headaches, nausea, vertigo, or discomfort in the abdomen. On rare occasions, they could result in more severe adverse effects such as allergic responses or liver damage.

Interactions with Other Drugs: Some antifungal medications, especially oral ones, may interact with other medicines to reduce their effectiveness or cause negative side effects. It's critical to let your doctor know about all your prescriptions.

Resistance Development: Excessive or improper use of antifungal medications might result in Candida resistance, which makes treating infections in the future more difficult.

Over-the-counter and prescription medications are useful in controlling the infection and reducing symptoms of vaginal candidiasis. For best effects and to prevent difficulties, it is important to be aware of their possible adverse effects and use them under a doctor's supervision.

Chapter Six

All-Natural and Integrative Therapies

Natural Treatments for Vaginal Candida

Several home remedies have been traditionally utilized to manage vaginal candidiasis for people looking for alternatives to conventional therapies. Even though some of these treatments might be helpful, it's crucial to use caution and evaluate their efficacy:

Yogurt: A common home cure involves applying plain, unsweetened yogurt straight to the vaginal area or taking it inside. Live cultures of Lactobacillus found in yogurt have the potential to suppress the growth of Candida by assisting in the restoration of the normal bacterial balance in the vagina.

Garlic: The antifungal qualities of garlic are well known. Some recommend leaving a peeled garlic clove in the vagina overnight, however, this can irritate the area. Adding more garlic to your diet or taking pills is a safer option.

Coconut Oil: Due to its antifungal qualities, coconut oil can be topically applied to afflicted areas to reduce inflammation and combat yeast infection. Make sure the oil is unrefined and organic to prevent any additives that can aggravate the skin even more.

Apple Cider Vinegar: It is said that putting a cup of apple cider vinegar in a warm bath will help balance the pH in the vagina and lessen yeast growth. It is not advised to apply directly to the vaginal region, though, since this may result in burning and discomfort.

Tea Tree Oil: Tea tree oil has potent antifungal qualities and can be administered externally after being diluted with a carrier oil (like coconut oil). Tea tree oil is strong and might irritate skin if it isn't diluted properly, so use caution while using it.

Although these therapies provide relief for certain women, they may not have the same effect on others. It's critical to keep an eye on symptoms and see a doctor if they get worse or continue. Certain over-the-counter medicines, especially those administered topically to the vaginal region, have the potential to irritate or trigger allergic reactions. Always start with a little patch of skin.

The Influence of Probiotics

Probiotics are good bacteria that can help maintain the general health of the vagina and stop yeast infections from coming back. There are various methods to incorporate these into your routine:

Probiotic Supplements: Taking oral probiotic supplements can help keep the balance of bacteria in the stomach and vagina healthy and may lower the risk of candidiasis. Particular strains to look for include Lactobacillus rhamnosus and Lactobacillus reuteri.

Yogurt and Fermented Foods: You may naturally increase your body's levels of good bacteria by including probiotic-rich foods like yogurt, kefir, sauerkraut, and kimchi in your diet.

Vaginal Probiotics: Certain products, such as probiotic suppositories, are made especially for vaginal use. These can be put into the vagina to stop Candida growth and immediately return the bacterial balance.

Taking probiotics regularly can help guard against recurrent illnesses. Probiotics enhance immune system performance, intestinal health, and general well-being in addition to supporting vaginal health.

Probiotics work best when taken continuously over an extended period. Although they are not a quick treatment, they may have long-term advantages.

It's advisable to speak with a healthcare professional before beginning any new supplement, particularly if you have any underlying medical concerns.

Herbal Remedies: Effective and Ineffective

Another natural method for treating vaginal candidiasis is the use of herbal medicines. Although several herbs have demonstrated potential, others are either unsupported by science or potentially dangerous:

Boric Acid: Recurrent yeast infections have been treated with vaginally inserted boric acid capsules. It works especially well against Candida strains that don't respond well to conventional antifungal therapies. But boric acid should only be used as prescribed because it might be harmful if swallowed.

Goldenseal: Berberine, an alkaloid having antifungal qualities, is found in goldenseal. As a supplement, it can be used orally to help fight Candida overgrowth. Its usefulness, particularly for vaginal candidiasis, hasn't been thoroughly researched, nevertheless.

Aloe Vera: External application of aloe vera gel, renowned for its calming qualities, helps ease inflammation and itching. Although it doesn't deal with the yeast directly, it can help control symptoms.

Echinacea: Echinacea is frequently used as an immune system stimulant. Although it promotes general health and may help avoid infections, there is little proof that it directly combats Candida.

The quality and strength of herbal supplements can differ as they are not subject to the same regulations as prescription drugs. Select goods from reliable vendors. Certain herbs have the potential to have adverse effects or interact with medicines. It's crucial to speak with a doctor before beginning any natural remedy.

<u>Modifications to Diet and Lifestyle to Avoid Recurrence</u>

To prevent recurrence, dietary and lifestyle modifications are frequently necessary for the long-term therapy of vaginal candidiasis:

Reduce Sugar Intake: Candida is a sugar-feeding yeast, so cutting back on sugar-filled foods, processed carbs, and alcohol will help starve the yeast and stop it from growing.

Eat a Balanced Diet: Make sure you eat a diet high in fruits, vegetables, lean meats, and good fats. Consume a lot of fiber to promote gut health and preserve a healthy microbiota.

Wear Breathable Clothing: Avoid wearing tight clothing that might trap heat and moisture and instead choose loose-fitting, breathable cotton undergarments, which will encourage the growth of yeast.

Maintain Good Hygiene: Wash your genitalia with water and a light, unscented soap. Douching should be avoided since it may upset the vagina's normal bacterial balance.

Control Stress: Extended periods of stress can impair immunity and upset hormonal equilibrium, increasing vulnerability to infections. Include stress-relieving pursuits in your daily routine, such as physical activity, meditation, or hobbies.

Remain Hydrated: Drinking lots of water promotes general health, including vaginal health, and aids in the removal of toxins from the body.

The key to avoiding repeated infections is to implement these adjustments consistently. Long-term health advantages can result from the effort, even though it can take some time to experience the full effects. Since every person's body is unique, figuring out the food and lifestyle changes that suit you the best may require some trial and error.

Natural and holistic therapies, especially when combined with or added to traditional treatments, can be useful in controlling and avoiding vaginal candidiasis. You may maintain vaginal health and avoid recurring infections by taking a proactive strategy that incorporates home remedies, probiotics, herbal therapies, and lifestyle modifications.

Chapter Seven

Preventing Vaginal Candidiasis

Daily Habits to Maintain Vaginal Health

Maintaining daily habits that promote vaginal health is crucial for preventing vaginal candidiasis. These habits help create an environment that discourages yeast overgrowth and supports a healthy balance of bacteria:

Gently clean the vaginal area daily with warm water and mild, unscented soap. Avoid using harsh soaps, scented products, or douches, as they can disrupt the natural balance of bacteria and lead to irritation or infection.

Moisture creates an ideal environment for yeast to thrive. After bathing or swimming, make sure to dry the vaginal area thoroughly. Change out of wet swimsuits and sweaty workout clothes as soon as possible to prevent moisture buildup.

Incorporating probiotics into your daily routine, whether through supplements or fermented foods like yogurt and kefir, can help maintain a healthy vaginal microbiome and reduce the risk of yeast infections.

While antibiotics are sometimes necessary, they can disrupt the balance of bacteria in the vagina, leading to yeast overgrowth. Use antibiotics only when prescribed and take the full course as directed by your healthcare provider.

Wear cotton underwear and avoid synthetic materials that trap heat and moisture. Cotton allows the skin to breathe and helps keep the vaginal area dry.

Tips for a Yeast-Free Diet

Diet plays a significant role in preventing vaginal candidiasis. Making mindful food choices can help you avoid yeast overgrowth and maintain a healthy balance in your body:

Reduce Sugar and Refined Carbohydrates: Candida feeds on sugar, so cutting down on sugary foods, sweets, and refined carbohydrates like white bread and pasta can help starve the yeast and prevent overgrowth.

-Incorporate Anti-Fungal Foods: Certain foods have natural antifungal properties that can help combat Candida. These include garlic, coconut oil, ginger, and apple cider vinegar. Regularly incorporating these into your diet can support your body's defense against yeast infections.

Eat Fermented Foods: Fermented foods like yogurt, sauerkraut, kimchi, and kefir are rich in probiotics that support a healthy gut and vaginal microbiome. Regular consumption can help maintain the balance of good bacteria, reducing the likelihood of yeast infections.

Stay Hydrated: Drinking plenty of water is essential for overall health, including vaginal health. Proper hydration helps flush out toxins and supports the body's natural detoxification processes, which can help prevent yeast overgrowth.

Balance Your Diet with Fiber: A diet rich in fiber supports a healthy digestive system and helps prevent blood sugar spikes, which can contribute to yeast overgrowth. Include plenty of vegetables, whole grains, and legumes in your diet.

The Importance of Hygiene and Proper Clothing

Good hygiene and appropriate clothing choices are key to preventing vaginal candidiasis. These practices help reduce the risk of moisture buildup and irritation, both of which can contribute to yeast infections:

Avoid Irritating Products: Steer clear of scented tampons, pads, sprays, and bubble baths, as they can irritate the vaginal area and disrupt the natural pH balance. Opt for unscented, hypoallergenic products instead.

Change Sanitary Products Regularly: During menstruation, change tampons and pads regularly to keep the area clean and dry. Prolonged use of the same product can create a breeding ground for bacteria and yeast.

Wear Loose-Fitting Clothing: Tight clothing, especially around the genital area, can trap moisture and create a warm environment that encourages yeast growth. Opt for loose-fitting pants, skirts, and breathable fabrics.

Choose Natural Fabrics: Natural fabrics like cotton, linen, and bamboo are breathable and help wick moisture away from the skin. Avoid synthetic materials like nylon and polyester, which can trap heat and moisture.

Sleep Without Underwear: Giving your body a break from underwear at night allows the vaginal area to breathe and reduces the risk of moisture buildup. Sleeping without underwear can be particularly beneficial for those prone to yeast infections.

<u>Managing Stress and Its Impact on Vaginal Health</u>

Stress has a significant impact on overall health, including vaginal health. Chronic stress can weaken the immune system, disrupt hormonal balance, and make the body more susceptible to infections, including vaginal candidiasis:

Practice Stress-Reduction Techniques: Incorporate stress-reducing activities into your daily routine, such as meditation, deep breathing exercises, yoga, or mindfulness. These practices can help calm the mind and body, reducing the impact of stress on your health.

Stay Physically Active: Regular physical activity is a powerful stress reliever. Exercise releases endorphins, which are natural mood boosters, and helps reduce stress hormones like cortisol. Aim for at least 30 minutes of moderate exercise most days of the week.

Get Adequate Sleep: Quality sleep is essential for managing stress and maintaining a healthy immune system. Aim for 7-9 hours of sleep per night to allow your body to rest, recover, and stay resilient against infections.

Maintain a Balanced Routine: A balanced routine that includes time for work, relaxation, and hobbies can help manage stress levels. Overworking or neglecting self-care can lead to burnout and increased stress, which may impact your vaginal health.

Seek Support When Needed: Don't hesitate to seek support from friends, family, or a mental health professional if you're feeling overwhelmed by stress. Talking about your concerns and finding healthy coping mechanisms can make a significant difference in managing stress.

Preventing vaginal candidiasis requires a combination of good hygiene, proper clothing choices, a balanced diet, and effective stress management. By adopting these habits and making mindful lifestyle choices, you can reduce the risk of yeast infections and support long-term vaginal health.

Chapter Eight

Special Considerations

Pregnancy-Related Vaginal Candidiasis

Significant hormonal changes that occur during pregnancy may raise the risk of vaginal candidiasis. Pregnancy-related elevated estrogen levels can create an environment that encourages Candida overgrowth Because greater amounts of estrogen can cause an increase in glycogen, a form of sugar, in the vaginal tissues, pregnant women are more vulnerable to yeast infections. This sugar gives Candida an abundance of food, which causes an overgrowth.

It's critical to select medical interventions that are safe for the mother and the growing fetus during pregnancy. Topical antifungal creams and suppositories, including miconazole or clotrimazole, are often advised and regarded as safe. Fluconazole and other oral antifungal drugs are generally avoided because of the possible dangers to the unborn child.

Before beginning any vaginal candidiasis treatment, expectant mothers should always speak with their healthcare practitioner. To ensure appropriate therapy and rule out other possible infections, a precise diagnosis is essential. By wearing breathable cotton pants, practicing excellent genital hygiene, and avoiding douches or scented products that could upset the pH balance in the vagina, pregnant women can lower their risk of developing yeast infections.

Menopause and Yeast Infections

Another stage of life where hormonal changes may impact vaginal health and raise the risk of vaginal candidiasis is menopause. The drop in estrogen levels that occurs during menopause can cause modifications to the vaginal environment, such as a thinning of the walls and a reduction in the natural acidity that guards against infections. The vaginal region may become more prone to yeast infections as a result of these modifications.

Vaginal candidiasis in menopausal women can cause burning, itching, and unusual discharge, just like in younger women. However, a correct diagnosis is crucial because these symptoms can occasionally be mistaken for other menopausal changes. During menopause, yeast infections can be effectively managed with over-the-counter and prescription antifungal medications.

Hormone replacement treatment (HRT) can help women who have recurrent infections by boosting vaginal health and estrogen levels. HRT isn't appropriate for everyone, so it's best to speak with a healthcare professional about it.

Vaginal Moisturisers and Lubricants: Using these products will help lessen the irritation that may lead to yeast infections and relieve vaginal dryness, a typical problem during menopause.

Handling Vaginal Candida in Women with Diabetes

Because diabetes can raise blood sugar levels, which can encourage Candida growth, diabetic women are more likely to develop vaginal candidiasis. Women with diabetes who have high blood sugar levels may be more susceptible to yeast overgrowth. The vaginal fluids may contain sugar, which would give Candida something to eat.

Recurrent yeast infections can be avoided by properly controlling blood sugar levels. To lower their risk of Candida overgrowth, women with diabetes should collaborate closely with their healthcare physician to maintain ideal blood glucose levels.

Women with diabetes may need more extensive or prolonged therapy to cure vaginal candidiasis. Antifungal medications applied topically and taken orally can also be beneficial, but managing blood sugar is essential to avoiding recurrence.

To maintain a healthy vaginal microbiota, diabetic women can consider adding probiotics to their diet, wearing breathable clothing, and practicing excellent vaginal hygiene in addition to controlling their blood sugar.

Sexual health and partner treatment

Sexual partners may occasionally contract vaginal candidiasis from one another, which can result in recurring infections. Effective therapy and prevention of yeast infections require addressing the components of sexual health that are affected by them. Even if a woman's sexual partner is asymptomatic, treating them both may be essential if she has recurrent vaginal candidiasis. This is especially crucial when the illness returns soon after therapy. A medical professional can suggest suitable treatment plans for both partners.

Since sexual activity can irritate the vaginal tissues and possibly transmit the infection, it is typically advised to refrain from sexual activity while receiving therapy for vaginal candidiasis. When engaging in sexual activity, wearing a condom might lessen the chance of irritation and transmission.

Preventing the transmission of yeast infections and lowering the chance of recurrence can be achieved by adhering to appropriate sexual health practices, such as using condoms and making sure both partners receive treatment when needed.

Managing vaginal candidiasis and preserving general sexual health need an open conversation with a sexual partner regarding symptoms, treatment, and preventive actions.

Unique factors including diabetes, menopause, pregnancy, and sexual health are important to take into account when managing and preventing vaginal candidiasis. Comprehending the distinct obstacles and therapeutic alternatives linked to these variables may assist females in making knowledgeable choices and preserving their vaginal well-being across various life phases.

Chapter Nine

When to Get Expert Assistance

While many women can treat mild cases of vaginal candidiasis at home or with over-the-counter medications, there are occasions when seeking professional medical attention is necessary. Understanding the warning indications that home remedies might not be adequate is essential for your well-being.

See a doctor if symptoms like burning, itching, or strange discharge don't go away after trying over-the-counter medication or home remedies. Extended symptoms may point to a new kind of infection entirely, a more serious infection, or a Candida strain that is resistant.

Recurrent vaginal candidiasis is defined as having more than four yeast infections in a calendar year.

To address the underlying reasons for recurrent infections, a more thorough evaluation and long-term treatment plan may be necessary. This plan may typically involve prescription medication or lifestyle modifications.

You should see a doctor if you suffer from severe symptoms, which include extreme itching, noticeable swelling, or extreme redness.

These symptoms may indicate an adverse reaction to medications or a more serious ailment. Pregnancy, diabetes, or a compromised immune system are a few circumstances that might make vaginal candidiasis more difficult to treat. To guarantee that the infection is treated successfully and securely in these situations, expert assistance is required.

It's best to contact a healthcare practitioner for a proper diagnosis if you're not sure if your symptoms are caused by a yeast infection or something else (such as bacterial vaginosis or a sexually transmitted infection). A misdiagnosis may result in ineffective treatment, exacerbating existing problems, or extending agony.

How to Have a Successful Conversation with Your Healthcare Professional

Having good communication with your physician is essential to getting the best treatment possible. Here are some tips for maximizing the value of your doctor's visit:

Jot down all of your symptoms, including when they first appeared, how bad they are, and any remedies you've tried, before your consultation. Make a note of any additional medical illnesses you may have as well as any medications you are taking, as they may affect your options for therapy.

Even if your symptoms are humiliating, make sure to explain them to your healthcare practitioner in detail. Vaginal health is a common concern, and to properly diagnose and treat you, your provider needs precise information.

If there is anything your provider says that you don't understand, don't be afraid to ask questions. Whether it's about the diagnosis, treatment options, or potential side effects, asking questions ensures you're fully educated about your health.

Enquire about all available treatment alternatives, as well as the advantages and disadvantages of each. In particular, if you have a preference for one treatment over another, this covers both traditional and alternative therapies.

Talk with your clinician about any recurrent infections you may have had. Managing your health requires discussing long-term preventive measures and comprehending the potential causes of recurrence.

Expectations for a Medical Examination

A medical examination for vaginal candidiasis typically consists of a few essential steps and is fairly simple. It can make you feel more at ease to know what to anticipate during the process:

Your doctor will begin by enquiring about your medical background, current symptoms, and previous treatments that you have tried. They might also enquire about your cleanliness habits, sexual health, and other matters that might have an impact on the health of your vagina.

The medical professional will examine the vaginal region physically to look for any symptoms of infection, such as redness, swelling, or discharge. To get a better view, this might entail gently opening the vagina with a speculum. The healthcare professional may use a cotton swab to collect a sample of vaginal discharge to confirm the diagnosis. Typically, a lab receives this sample to determine whether Candida is present and to rule out other infections.

Depending on your situation, the doctor can suggest more blood work to rule out any underlying diseases like diabetes or compromised immune systems that might be causing your symptoms. Your physician will go over the diagnosis and suggest a course of treatment following the examination and tests. This could involve lifestyle modifications, prescription antifungal drugs, or additional testing if necessary.

If you are receiving a longer-term treatment plan or have experienced recurrent infections, your provider may arrange a follow-up appointment to assess your progress. During follow-up appointments, be sure to note any new or worsening symptoms.

The key to successfully managing vaginal candidiasis is understanding when to seek professional assistance. You can make sure that you obtain the greatest care for your health by being aware of the warning indications that your home remedies might not be sufficient, communicating with your healthcare provider effectively, and knowing what to expect from a medical checkup.

Chapter Ten

Long-Term Strategies for Living Without Yeast

Sustaining Vaginal Health Following Therapy

It's critical to concentrate on preserving vaginal health once vaginal candidiasis has been effectively treated to avoid recurrent infections. By putting these tactics into practice, you can support Candida's control and long-term well-being by Including probiotics in your diet regularly by consuming foods like kefir, sauerkraut, and yogurt or by taking supplements. Probiotics have a critical role in preserving the proper balance of bacteria in the vagina and gut, which inhibits the growth of yeast.

Avoid sugar and processed carbs as much as possible because they can feed Candida and encourage its growth. Instead, follow a balanced diet. Prioritise whole foods, a diet high in fruits and vegetables, lean proteins, and healthy fats. Exercise regularly to strengthen your immune system and preserve your general well-being.

Infections can be triggered by stress, which is another thing that exercise helps address.

Wash the area with water and mild, unscented soap to maintain proper vaginal hygiene. Steer clear of perfumed and douching products since they may upset the vagina's natural pH balance.

Steer clear of tight-fitting apparel that can retain heat and moisture, and opt instead for undergarments made of natural fibers like cotton. Venturing the space aids in preventing the conditions that allow yeast to proliferate.

Recurrence Prevention: Advice and Techniques

Being proactive with your health is key to preventing the recurrence of vaginal candidiasis. Here are some useful hints and techniques to prevent yeast infections:

Monitor Blood Sugar Levels: Controlling your blood sugar levels is essential to preventing yeast overgrowth if you have diabetes or insulin resistance. To properly manage your disease, collaborate with your healthcare practitioner.

Strengthen Your Immune System: Your best line of defense against recurring infections is a robust immune system. Keep up a healthy lifestyle by practicing stress reduction, eating a diet high in nutrients, exercising frequently, and getting enough sleep.

Be Aware of Your Medications: Some drugs, such as oral contraceptives and antibiotics, can upset the delicate bacterial balance in the vagina and cause yeast infections. Talk to your healthcare practitioner about alternate drugs or preventive actions if you are susceptible to candidiasis.

Remain Hydrated: Drinking lots of water promotes good health throughout the body and aids in the removal of toxins, which lowers the risk of infections.

Practice Safe Sex: To lower the chance of spreading illnesses between partners, use condoms when engaging in sexual activity. If you or your significant other frequently have yeast infections, think about getting treatment together to stop reinfection.

Avoid Triggers: Recognise and steer clear of situations where wearing tight clothing, wet swimsuits for extended periods, or strong detergents could result in yeast infections. The likelihood of a recurrence can be greatly decreased by being aware of these factors.

Aspects of Coping with Chronic Infections on an Emotional and Psychological Level

Having recurrent vaginal candidiasis can be detrimental to your mental and physical health. It's critical to recognize these difficulties and develop coping mechanisms:

Having a persistent infection can cause anxiety, shame, or irritation. It's critical to acknowledge these feelings and recognize that they are a normal reaction to managing a recurrent medical condition.

If you need emotional help, don't be afraid to ask friends, family, or support groups for it. Talking to someone who can relate to your experiences can be consoling and help you feel less alone.

Information gives you power. Your sense of control over vaginal candidiasis will increase with your knowledge of the condition and how to treat it. This might ease your anxiety and boost your self-assurance in your ability to take care of your health.

Prolonged stress can impair immunity and increase the likelihood that infections will return. Use mindfulness exercises to reduce stress and enhance your general mental well-being, such as yoga, meditation, or deep breathing.

You should think about seeing a mental health professional if you discover that managing chronic infections is seriously lowering your quality of life. Counseling can offer helpful strategies for handling the psychological effects of recurring medical conditions.

Prioritize your well-being by doing things that make you happy and calm. Self-care practices, such as reading a book, having a warm bath, or going outside, can help you feel better.

Maintaining a yeast-free lifestyle necessitates a continuous focus on lifestyle decisions, preventative measures, and emotional health in addition to treating infections as they appear. You may improve your quality of life, preserve vaginal health, and stop recurrence by implementing these long-term strategies.

Conclusion

Final Thoughts

We've covered all the ins and outs of vaginal candidiasis in this guide, arming you with the knowledge you need to recognize, treat, and avoid this prevalent illness. The main ideas we discussed are as follows:

First, we clarified what vaginal candidiasis is and how it differs from other vaginal illnesses like bacterial vaginosis. We studied the science of Candida overgrowth and the factors that lead to infection in the vaginal environment.

We outlined the typical signs of vaginal candidiasis and offered advice on how to distinguish them from other infections. We also talked about when it's imperative to get medical attention.

We looked at nutrition, lifestyle, and several drugs as well as other factors that lead to Candida overgrowth. We also discussed the difficulties in treating recurrent infections and the significance of comprehending their underlying causes.

We talked about how to diagnose vaginal candidiasis, including how to use at-home test kits and how crucial it is to get a professional medical examination. A precise diagnosis is essential for successful treatment.

We went over the advantages and disadvantages of both conventional and natural treatments in great depth. We underlined the significance of selecting the best strategy for your particular needs, whether it be through over-the-counter drugs, prescription therapies, or complementary therapies.

We provided advice on nutrition, hygiene, and lifestyle modifications as well as techniques for preserving vaginal health and averting recurrence. Particular attention was also given to various life periods, including pregnancy and menopause.

We covered when seeing a doctor is essential as well as how to interact with them during appointments. Getting the greatest care possible is ensured when you know when to ask for assistance.

Lastly, we spoke about long-term methods of avoiding yeast, such as the psychological and emotional ramifications of managing persistent infections. We underlined the value of assistance and self-care in preserving general well-being.

Although vaginal candidiasis can be an annoying and inconvenient illness, you can take charge of your health and avoid further infections if you have the correct information and resources. You now have the knowledge you need to better understand your body, choose a course of action, and lead a lifestyle that promotes long-term vaginal health thanks to this book.

Never forget that you are not traveling alone. Seeking help—from loved ones, support groups, or healthcare providers—can make a big impact on women who experience comparable issues. You should prioritize your health, and by acting now, you can make tomorrow healthier and more comfortable.

As you proceed, keep learning, pay attention to your body, and speak out for your health. Your efforts to recognize and treat candidiasis are admirable and empowering, regardless of whether you're managing a single bout of the illness or persistent infections.

Additional Reading and Supporting Resources

Here are some more resources that may be useful as you continue on your path to improved vaginal health:

Book: Take into consideration reading more in-depth books about women's health, especially those that address holistic medicine, nutrition, and vaginal health.

Websites: Reputable medical websites with a wealth of information on vaginal health and related subjects include the Mayo Clinic, WebMD, and the American College of Obstetricians and Gynaecologists (ACOG).

Support Groups: You can ask questions, share stories, and find solace in the knowledge that you're not alone by joining online communities and support groups. Women can discuss candidiasis and other health issues in forums, Facebook groups, and on websites like Reddit.

Medical Professionals: Stay in constant contact with your medical professional. They can provide you with individualized guidance, confidently guide you through your health journey, and refer specialists if necessary.

To sum up, keeping your general health depends on your dedication to knowing about vaginal candidiasis and managing it. Remind yourself that your health is important and that you should always take preventative measures